The Friendly Bacteria:

A guide to the friendly flora in your gut

Introduction on how to keep you gut healthy, and recipes for bacteria-friendly foods

Eve Bell

Table of Contents

Disclaimer

While all attempts have been made to verify the information provided in this book, the author does assume any responsibility for errors, omissions, or contrary interpretations of the subject matter contained within. The information provided in this book is for educational and entertainment purposes only. The reader is responsible for his or her own actions and the author does not accept any responsibilities for any liabilities or damages, real or perceived, resulting from the use of this information.

The trademarks that are used are without any consent, and the publication of the trademark is without permission or backing by the trademark owner. All trademarks and brands within this book are for clarifying purposes only and are the owned by the owners themselves, not affiliated with this document.

Bacteria

From our early years, we've been informed that bacteria are responsible for causing illnesses. As a result, our parents endeavored to maintain surfaces free of potential threats to our health. As you grew older, you found yourself questioning why you were advised to consume yogurt alongside antibiotic prescriptions. As it turns out, there are beneficial bacteria in your small intestine that contribute to gut and digestive health. Seeking more information online, you encountered an overwhelming array of websites and sources that made your eyes glaze over. You've been in search of a comprehensive manual detailing all the beneficial bacteria in your gut and their advantages. Well, look no further—this guide is tailored just for you!

Acididophi - what is?

You've purchased this book to answer the questions your mind keeps generating on the friendly flora in your digestive system. You've seen the names of some of them on milk jugs in grocery stores and on supplements in health food stores but have too been apprehensive to ask questions to learn more about them. This book has been formatted to teach you:

• The different friendly bacteria in your gut and their purpose.

• The things that can cause an imbalance in your gut.

• How having a healthy gut can keep your immune system strong.

• Who fermented foods can help with the colonies in your gut and keep them healthy.

• Recipes on how to make fermented foods.

• Supplements you can purchase which can also help maintain the balance in your gut.

So, if you're looking to learn more about your body and keeping it healthy, swipe the page and let's get started!

Chapter 1 - The Friendly Bacteria

There are bacteria in your small intestine that aids in the digestive process. You've probably only heard of two types, Lactobacillus and Bifidobacterium. There more sub species of those two and a few more.

Lactobacillus Species

L. Acidophilus-This is one of the most talked about stains of the species. It may even be the most important strain. It is the strain responsible for overall digestive health and nutrient absorption. Acidophilus also gives relief from cramping, diarrhea, and flatulence. It promotes immune system health and also helps maintain balance in women's urinary and vaginal health.

L. Fermentum- This is found in probiotic foods like sourdough and kimchi. Fermentum produces two superoxides: dismutase and glutathione. These antioxidants help to neutralize toxins in the small intestine, making this strain of bacteria important when you detoxify your system and in the digestive process.

L. Plantarum- This strain is known for being able to produce hydrogen peroxide in the body. Once produced, this compound defends against harmful bacteria in food, preventing indigestion and possibly some cases of food poisoning. Plantarum is also an immune system booster.

L. Rhamnosus- This probiotic is very resilient, being able to survive traveling through the GI tract. Because of this, Rhamnosus is a boon for vaginal health. It's also instrumental in helping people overcome, and in some cases prevent, Traveler's Diarrhea.

L. Salivarius- This probiotic is known for growing in the most hostile of places. It loves high salt or no oxygen environments. You can find it in the mouth, throat and even your sinuses. Salivarius also helps stop the growth of aggressive bacteria. It can promote oral health and boost the immune system.

L. Paracasei- When you're looking for a probiotic strain to lower pH and improve liver function, Paracasei is that very strain. It is resistant to stomach acid when taken with casein (milk protein).

L. Gasseri- This is a recently discovered strain of probiotic. It has been found to be linked to the flora in the vagina, making it good for vaginal health as a whole. When taken in combination with B. Longum, it can help with occasional diarrhea.

L. Reuteri grows in the oral cavity and the intestine. It is used to boost oral health, immune health, and digestion as a whole.

Bifidobacterium Species

B. Bifidum- This is the first probiotic strain that most people think of when looking for friendly bacteria to promote digestive health, and it may very well be one of the most important. It is a great promoter of digestive health; it helps the body to absorb nutrients from food and drink, and also helps with diarrhea related to travel. It can help regulate the growth of detrimental bacteria, molds, and yeasts. This is one of the probiotics that can help prevent Candida.

B. Longum- This *bifidobacteria* can help the system breakdown carbohydrates and neutralize gut toxins.
It also scavenges free radicals, which helps to keep the immune system functioning properly. It helps to maintain healthy digestion and helps during the detoxing process.

B. Infantis- Named such because it is found more prevalent in babies; this strain decreases as we age. It helps prevent bloating and constipation.

Bacillus Species

B. Coagulans- This strain helps the body process calcium and the body's abilities to use it properly as well as phosphorus and iron. It helps the stomach by helping to stir gastric juices to action. It even helps with pH level of the vagina.

Streptococcus Species

Surprisingly enough, there are strains of these bacteria that are good for your body and actually live in your body.

S. Salivarius K12- Found in the mucus membranes of the mouth, it helps to make substances that prevent detrimental bacteria from forming. Testing has proven to reduce the number of sore throats, and promoted ear health as well as reduce plaque scores.

S. Salivarius M18- This is a strain that promotes the health of teeth and gums.

Chapter 2 - Friendly Bacteria and Diseases

We've covered all the friendly bacteria in your gut and what they help with in terms of immune system and other system health, but what happens when the balance is off, and you don't have the levels of healthy bacteria you need to prevent diseases and other issues?

Candida Albicans

Believe it or not, this is already in your system. It's just not at large enough levels to be considered overgrowth. Most would equate Candida as a vaginal yeast infection, but it is also known as thrush (mouth yeast), and can also be located on the skin and in the respiratory system.

This is the most commonly known condition that occurs when the gut is not in balance. There are three causes:

• Antibiotics, the prescribed kind, do not discriminate between the bacteria that is supposed to be in your gut and the bacterial infection that has taken up residence in your body. This means, it kills everything, including the probiotics listed in the previous chapter. Killing too many leaves the growth of Candida unchecked, leading to yeast infections.

• A sugar and yeast heavy diet can also contribute to Candida running rampant. Avoiding processed foods and lowering your intake of yeasty foods can help keep your gut at healthy levels.

• Stress, this seems to show up in every list of causes to virtually every disease known to man, but it is also one of the main contributing factors. It can cause imbalances which lead to inflammation of the gut as well as Candida.

This imbalance can happen in men and women.

Symptoms

There are some things to look for if you may suspect you have Candida overgrowth, but, as always, to make sure, go to your doctor. Here are some of the more prevalent symptoms.

• Cravings for sugar and carbs - I don't mean the occasional "I feel like having 'x'." I mean you *have* to have it to the point where most of what you purchase has to have either sugar or be high in carbohydrates. This is because Candida loves sugar and will do anything to you to ingest more. It also thrives off of yeast.

• Tired, lack of energy, fatigued-No matter what you do, you just can't seem to get in gear to do *any*thing. It doesn't matter if take naps or get plenty of rest. You're still ready to back to sleep and just not motivated to do even everyday tasks and errands.

• You may either gain weight or find it hard to lose weight.

• You are irritable, anxious when you're not normally so, or are having feelings of depression.

• Annoying skin problems you've never had before.

• Constant stomach problems

- Food allergies you haven't had before.

- Constant headaches

- Asthma

- Worse than normal PMS

- IBS

- If you are a female, you may experience a thick milky discharge, yellow patches in the mouth, urination that burns, and vaginal itching. If you do, don't wait to see your doctor as this can become a more severe condition called Candidemia (when the Candida enters the bloodstream).

How to Treat It

The best way to treat Candida is to avoid the following foods for a few weeks:

Sugary foods, starches, mold, yeast, high fructose corn syrup, regular syrup, alcohol, vinegar, breads, carrots, potatoes, peanuts, corn, mushrooms, milk, aged cheeses, citrus fruits, soda, and highly processed foods.

I know these sounds like a very restrictive diet, but it will give your body the best possible chance to get Candida under control. Stick to fresh vegetables, meats, eggs, seeds, nuts, olive oil, extra virgin coconut oil, water, and herbal tea.

Exercise gets the body moving in the right direction as well in order to get the Candida back to normal.

Avoiding stress in this world is not possible, but it is important to keep stress levels at a minimum. Here are a few things you can do to manage your stress:

• Sit and listen to soothing music, jazz and classical come to mind here. Just close your eyes and get lost in the music. Any music that relaxes you will be of benefit to you.

• Read a book. Sit down and pick a book, not a Kindle or Nook, an actual book and read it. Lose yourself in the story.

• Take a soothing bath. You can add mineral salts to the bath, light candles, and play music while in the bath. Some people even read in the bath.

• Unplug when you get home and just do something that does not require the computer or your cell phone. Cook, dance, take up a hobby, anything that takes your mind of every day stresses will help you manage stress.

• Stop sweating the small stuff. In this world, the only person and situations you can control are you and whether you choose to be in those situations. Don't let little things bother you. If it isn't something that will largely affect your health, don't sweat it.

• Close your eyes; take a slow, deep breath in, and a slow, deep breath out. Repeat this about five times. You will feel calmer.

Probiotics

Eating kefir, yogurt, and fermented foods during your Candida period can help immensely in getting that yeast under control.

You can even purchase kefir grains online. I will get that a little later in the book.

Leaky Gut

This is another disease related to an imbalance in your gut. This steams from a severe case of Candida when the overgrowth creates roots, or hyphae, which creates holes in the bowel walls. These holes let harmful bacteria, microorganisms, and macromolecules pass through to the circulatory system. This is how this condition gets the name *Leaky Gut*. This illness can lead to more serious ones such as:

- Rheumatoid Arthritis,
- Arthritis that affects the spine (Akylosing Spondylitis),
- Multiple Sclerosis,
- Eczema,
- Fibromyalgia,
-Crohn's disease,
- Raynaud's Phenomenon,
- Chronic Urticaria (hives), and
- Inflammatory Bowel Disease.

All of the above are more commonly known as conditions of Irritable Bowel Syndrome.

Some of the major's symptoms of Leaky Gut are:

- Face swelling when taking in pungent odors.
- After eating you experience cramping and other signs of flatulence, like bloating.
- Your bowels switching between being constipated and having diarrhea.
- Headaches, not being able to concentrate, being irritable.
- Allergies to food you didn't have before.

Your bowel lining will become inflamed. There are some things that can trigger this:

- Taking prescribed hormones or corticosteroids.
- Overusing antibiotics.
- Having a diet heavy in processed foods.
- Increasing your carbohydrate intake.
- Increasing the amount of caffeine and alcoholic drinks.

You can already see a lot of similarities between suffering from Candida Albicans and Leaky Gut. There is a definite link between the two. This is why you have to maintain a healthy diet and learn to manage the stress in your life. A healthy diet and incorporating exercise can help keep the Candida in your system at healthy levels. It is a balance you can't afford to irritate.

Chapter 3 - Bacteria and Your Weight

Don't look at this section as a diet plan. Diets are temporary plans designed to help you lose weight in a short period of time. In order to have weight loss last, you have to make the commitment to changing how you eat, what you eat, and being more active every day. It's a lifestyle change, meaning it lasts for the rest of your life. So, you have to make decisions you are comfortable and can live with. This will make it a breeze to follow your new, healthier life. Here are some alternatives and suggestions for your new lifestyle:

Incorporate Raw Foods

This may take some digging on your part, but start adding raw foods to your diet. Start with salads and delve a little more into it. Make about 20% of your diet raw. This should help start you on your gut issues and put you on the road to a healthy weight.

Paleo

This type of diet prohibits the intake of processed foods and refined foods, like white sugar. It also has you avoiding grains, yeast, potatoes, and refined oils. Think of it as a carbohydrate-free, whole foods plan. With the amount of nut flours available, you shouldn't have a problem. There are plenty of websites and message boards you can look at to get some good recipes to add to your food plans.

Vegan

I am very reserved when recommended this type of diet. There are many websites out there that recommend this type of diet for people with Candida and other gut issues, but without meat, you will deficient in vitamin B-12, iron, and many essential amino acids. If you do want to leave out red meat, that is perfectly fine, but be careful with your fish and only purchase fresh fish or wild-caught frozen fish.

Organic Foods

Produce grown without chemical pesticides are your best bet, but don't be taken in and buy nothing but organic. If the produce you are looking at has a thick skin, you won't have to worry about the pesticides soaking through the skin into the meat of produce. This will save you a ton of money.

Fermented Foods

These are a definite must to add to your diet. They will help you immensely with maintaining the balance of friendly bacteria in your gut. Germany and Korea have a long tradition of eating fermented foods, Germany being sauerkraut and Korea with Kimchi. Why fermented foods?

These foods are prepared using lacto fermentation, the process where bacteria consume starches and sugars present in foods. This type of preparation helps preserve food, creates enzymes, B-vitamins, Omega-3 fatty acids, and of course, probiotics. Over the years, the practice of making fermented foods have fallen by the wayside to highly processed foods, fast foods, and other unhealthy ways of eating.

Chapter 4 - Fermented Foods and You

There are several recipes out there for you to try out, from drinks to yogurt and everything in-between.

Kombucha Tea - The Immortal Health Elixir

This is a fermented tea that has been used, and still is used, in China for centuries. It starts with a special tea that is sweetened and fermented by bacteria and yeast with a symbiotic relationship. It has only recently gained popularity in the Western World. This is due to the extensive research done in Russia and Germany to order to substantiate the claims that it can prevent or cure cancer, help with forms of arthritis and other prevalent diseases. They were not only able to back the claims, but also narrow down what exactly contributes to kombucha's benefits.
It was found to have high amounts of B-vitamins, antioxidants, and also glucaric acids, acids that inhibit the production of a cancer causing enzyme.

How to Make Your Own Kombucha Tea

First, you are going to need to need the started culture. You can get the live SCOBY (starter culture) online, or you can, if you prefer, get the dehydrated SCOBY online, too.

Tools you will need:

-Quart-Size Glass Jar, Mason jar is perfect
-Plastic or wooden spoon
-Coffee filter or cheesecloth
-Something to secure the cover to the jar. If you are using a Mason jar, it should have its own lid.

Ingredients you will need:

-2-3 Cups Purified water, this is water without fluoride or chlorine.
-1/4 Cup White sugar
-1 1/2 tsp loose tea/2 tea bags
-1/2 Cup Starter tea or Distilled White vinegar
-Active SCOBY

If you are using loose tea, be sure to remove the metal tea ball before adding the SCOBY.

1. Heat the water.
2. Add the sugar to the heated water.
3. Add the tea and let steep, 15-20 minutes. You can leave the tea in longer if you want a strong batch.
4. Cool to 68-85F.
5. Remove the tea bags, ball, or strain the loose tea if you did not use a tea ball.
6. Add starter tea. This is tea from another batch. If this is your first time, you can use distilled white vinegar.
7. Add the SCOBY
8. Cover the jar with either cheesecloth or the coffee filter and secure it with either the rim of the Mason jar lid or a rubber band.
9. Place it out of direct sunlight in room temperature for 7-30 days or until it has reached a desired taste. It's important to note that the longer you let it ferment, the more it will have a vinegar taste.
10. Pour the desired amount for drinking into a glass. Leave just enough to cover the SCOBY. This is the starter for the next batch.

How to Make Kefir

Many of you have seen this in stores in pretty packaging in the dairy section and wondered what it is. It is a beverage that has 200 times more live cultures than yogurt. It is a fermented drink that is normally made with raw milk, but can also be used with Coconut milk, rice milk, coconut water, and even goat's milk. Because it is fermented, most people who are lactose intolerant can drink the fermented cow milk with no problem.

Kefir is made with grains as a starter and has two different grains, milk and water grains. Each has their own way of being fermented.

Milk Kefir

Tools needed:
Same as for Kombucha, but you will need a plastic strainer to get the kefir grains out, and you will not need a tea bag or loose tea.

Ingredients you will need
1-2 tsp active Milk Kefir Grains
4 Cups of fresh milk, this would normally be raw milk.

How To Make Milk Kefir

1. Place the milk in the Mason jar

2. Add the grains

3. Cover with cheesecloth or coffee filter and secure with rubber band or Mason jar rim.

4. Leave at room temperature for about 24 hours. It will be faster in warmer temps. The milk will thicken.

5. Transfer the grains to a new jar of milk.

How to Make Coconut Milk Kefir

1. Place the milk grains in coconut milk. Use the amounts above.
2. Stir with a non-metal spoon.
3. Cover
4. Let sit at room temperature.
5. Start checking after 12 hours and remove grains once it is the thickness you want.

Water Kefir

Right off the bat, you will notice the difference in texture. These are clearer than the milk kefir. When this ferments, it will take on more soda qualities. You can use purified water or coconut water for this. Below is the recipe for purified water. You will need the same things you use for the milk kefir.

Ingredients
1 tsp water kefir grains
1 egg shell, cleaned with purified water to remove left-over egg
1 tbsp unsulfured molasses

How to make water kefir
1. Add the molasses to the water and shake until mixed
2. Add the egg shell

3. Add the grains

4. Cover

5. Let sit for 24 hours at room temperature

6. Strain out the water grains and transfer to another jar and make more.

You can also go online to find more recipes for your kefir. There are entire online communities dedicated to making, flavoring, and even trading grains.

Kimchi-Fermented Cabbage

Ingredients
10 Cups of water
2 Napa Cabbages washed and chopped into 2-inch squares
1 Cup coarse salt (sea salt preferred)
1 tbsp chopped garlic
1 tbsp chopped ginger
1/2 Cup red pepper flakes
2 tbsp sugar
5 scallions chopped into 1/2-inch pieces

How to Make it
1. In a glass bowl or non-metal pot, mix the salt into the water.
2. Place the cabbage in the water. Make sure all the leaves are under the water. Weight it down, if you have to.
3. Soak for 5 or 6 hours
4. In a separate bowl, mix the garlic, ginger, red pepper, sugar and scallions.
5. Take the cabbage out and rinse in cold water. Make sure to remove the excess liquid.
6. Coat the cabbage with the seasoning mix.
7. Pack it all in jar with a tight lid and allow fermenting for 2 to 3 days in a cool place.

Pickles

You see them in the stores and have even tried them, but have you ever wondered how to make them? Here is the simple way of doing it.

It makes two quarts:

Ingredients and tools

2 1-quart Mason/Ball Jars with lids, prepared according to manufacturer instructions.

3-1/2 lbs of medium cucumbers, which is about 14 of them

2 cups of water

1 cup white vinegar

1/4 Kosher Sill Pickle Mix (from the grocery store in the canning section)

1 deep stock pot

How to Make Them

1. Clean and scrub the cucumbers

2. Cut off the ends and make them into spears.

3. In a medium sauce pan, add the water vinegar, and dill pickle mix.

4. Heat water to a boil.

5. While the water is heating, pack the cucumber spears into the hot jars.

6. Ladle the liquid over the spears. Leave 1/2 inch between the liquid and the mouth of the jar. Using your finger tips, screw on the lids.

7. In the large stock pot, add regular water and begin to heat it.

8. Place the jars in the stock pot, making sure the lids are covered with the water.

9. Boil the jars for 15 minutes.

10. Take jars out of the pot and place them on the counter on a towel.

12. Check the seal after 24 hours. The button on the top of the jar should be down.

They will keep for up to a year.

Chapter 5 - Fermentation on the Go!

With our busy lives, some of us won't have the time to make pickles, kimchi or even sauerkraut. This is why you have to plan ahead and have things ready when you have to run errands or have more things to do in a day you don't know which way to turn.

Smoothies

If you want to start your morning with probiotics, but not take a bunch of pills, try this simple recipe:

1 Cup Vanilla Yogurt

1/4 Cup Almond Milk

2 Probiotic capsules

1 Cup of fruit of choice

Ice

1. Put the yogurt and milk in the blender on blend

2. Open the probiotic capsules and pour the contents into the blender.

3. Add the fruit and blend completely.

4. Add the ice to thicken.

If you have kefir made up, you can use that in place of the yogurt. Stores do sell kefir already made for convenience. This is perfect for when you're too busy to make it yourself.

Check your local store for sauerkraut. You can then take it home and place it in small containers to add to meals and for quick snacks.

Buyer Beware

There are some things you need to be aware of when buying probiotics. You've already got the list of them, but:

1. They need to be refrigerated. This helps them stay dormant long enough to travel through your system before they become active.

2. Know where the cultures come from. Do you research and be sure you're getting the best possible probiotics for your money.

Final tips

1. Take them on an empty stomach. This is one of the few times you will be told to take something on an empty stomach. This will help them get through your digestive system with a better chance at getting to their destination.

2. Start out with two in the morning. Like most natural supplements, you have to tailor them to your metabolism. Though every supplement comes with instructions, you have to take into account the recommended dose is for a person of average height and about 180 lbs. Once you start taking the supplement, wait a couple of weeks and take note of how your body is feeling. If you are feeling better, then the smallest dose is perfect for you. If not, add one more capsule at lunch and repeat the process.

3. You have to take the supplements for one week for each month you have had the symptoms. This is a baseline for how long it will take your system to heal itself with the aid of supplements. You didn't get sick overnight. It's only reasonable that you will not heal overnight either.

4. Check with a licensed Naturopath in your area to make sure you are on the right path to healing.

A Naturopath is a holistic physician that will work with you, body, mind and spirit, to make sure you will heal properly.

Conclusion

Taking care of your digestive system can be a chore or the easiest thing you have ever done to contribute to your well-being. You just need to listen to your body and learn what it's trying to tell you. I hope this book has helped you on the path to a better feeling, and more active, you.